BLOOMING THROUGH MENOPAUSE

ENJOYING THIS TIME OF LIFE WITH GRACE AND VIGOR THAT GOES BEYOND NUTRITIONAL GUIDELINES

Helen Clayton

Table of Content

Table of Content...3

Introduction..7

Understanding Menopause and it effects on diet 13

What is Menopause?.............................. 10

What is Perimenopause?........................10

Chapter One... 14

Nutritional needs during menopause............. 14

Fiber...15

Protein...15

Omega-3 Fatty Acids 16

Phytoestrogens...................................... 16

Water...17

Top Vitamins for Menopause 17

Chapter Two... 21

Foods to include in the Menopause diet......... 22

Protein: 22

Fatty fish:..23

Carbohydrates:.......................................23

Dairy and substitutes: 24

Fruits and vegetables:............................24

Beverages:..25

Other foods or supplements: 25

Snacks:... 26

Healthy Foods to consume during Menopause.. 27

Foods to avoid during Menopause.................31

Chapter Three...32

Hydration Importance.................................32
Why is it important to stay hydrated?........32
Signs of Dehydration:............................33
How much water should you drink to relieve menopausal symptoms and dehydration? 33
Avoiding dehydration during Menopause .34
Hydration can help reduce some menopause symptoms.............................35
Dehydration can worsen Some menopause symptoms..38
How to drink enough water during menopause...39
Exercise 40
Hot Weather...41
Illness or Other Health Concerns..............41
Which Fluids Are the Greatest for Hydration?...42
Which Beverages Need to be Avoided?...42
Chapter Four...**44**
Menopause diet meal plan.........................44
Menopausal weight loss:..........................44
Ideal diet plan for weight loss during Menopause...47
Weekly meal plan for weight loss during Menopause...50
Perimenopause diet plan to lose weight.........54
Chapter Five..**60**
Supplements for Menopausal women............60
Melatonin..61
Vitamin D and calcium............................62
Omega 3's...64

Magnesium..64

Phytoestrogens.. 65

Herbal remedies for Menopause 66

Black Cohosh... 67

St. John's Wort... 67

Wild yam.. 68

Dong Quai.. 69

Maca.. 69

Chapter Six.. **71**

Physical activity and its impacts....................71

Advantages of exercise............................71

Activities that can be beneficial.................72

Exercise Tips...74

Chapter Seven... **76**

Managing weight during Menopause..............76

Understanding Menopause and weight gain.
76

The relationship between Menopause and
weight gain..77

Common causes for weight gain during
Menopause.. 78

Menopausal weight gain's impact on health.
80

Techniques for Managing Weight Gain
During Menopause....................................82

Chapter Eight... **84**

Addressing specific symptoms.......................84

Hot flashes... 84

Vaginal infections problem 87

Irregular periods or bleeding..................... 89

Difficulty sleeping:.............................. 89

Memory issues:................................. 92

Urinary issues................................... 93

Mood swing:.................................... 94

Anxiety and depression:.........................97

Feelings regarding sex changing............. 98

Chapter Nine..101

Recipes for Menopause friendly meals........ 101

1.Salmon and Quinoa Bowl:...................101

2. Salad with Chickpeas and Spinach:....102

3. Tofu and Vegetable Stir-Fry.................104

4. Berries and Greek Yogurt Parfait........ 106

5. Avocado and Salmon Salad Wraps.....107

Conclusion.. 110

Introduction

"Blooming through Menopause" explores the complex relationship between nutrition and menopause which provides a thorough guidance to help you through this important stage of life with energy and wellbeing. Hormonal changes accompany women as they approach and through menopause, affecting both their physical and mental well-being. Acknowledging the significant impact of diet on these changes, this book emerges as a reliable guide, enabling readers to adopt a deliberate and methodical approach to eating throughout menopause.

The foundation is laid in the first few chapters, which go into the physiological subtleties of menopause and how the body responds to them. This section gives a comprehensive knowledge of the particular difficulties menopausal women confront, from shifting hormone levels to possible concerns about bone density. It establishes the foundational ideas of the menopausal diet by highlighting the significance of individualized dietary approaches for symptom relief and general health support.

As readers explore the nutritional needs during menopause, important components like calcium, vitamin D, and omega-3 fatty acids come into focus. The book helps readers make well-informed dietary decisions that will support hormonal balance, cardiovascular health, and bone health. The story is skillfully interwoven with useful advice on how to include phytoestrogens and other vital nutrients in everyday meals.

The book "Blooming through Menopause" places a strong emphasis on maintaining balance. The sections on foods to eat in moderation and foods to avoid or limit offer a road map for creating an equilibrium-promoting diet. Antioxidant-rich fruits and vegetables, lean proteins, and whole grains take center stage in the diet plan, while processed and sugary foods have a measured place.

The Importance of hydration—which is sometimes overlooked but yet vital—is highlighted, highlighting how water promotes general wellness. In addition to promoting mindful eating, the book stresses the significance of preserving appropriate fluid balance during this period of transformation.

The book's final sections include advice on meal planning, suggest supplements, and provide insights into properly managing weight while emphasizing practical implementation. Menopausal woman-specific recipes offer a delicious investigation of savory and nutrient-dense meals, bridging the gap between theory and reality.

"Blooming through Menopause" is more than just a cookbook; it's a comprehensive lifestyle partner that enables women to face this stage of life with fortitude, knowledge, and a revitalized feeling of wellbeing. The road towards improved health, vigor, and a balanced approach to eating during the menopausal transition begins as the reader turns the pages.

Understanding Menopause and it effects on diet

What is Menopause?

Menopause is feared by many women, who may regard it as a disease, catastrophe, or medical emergency. However, it's a typical, organic change that occurs as women age, much like puberty. The only exception is medical menopause, which happens following ovarian surgery, in certain cases of autoimmune illnesses, and as a result of certain cancer treatments.

The term "menopause" refers to the period of time that follows the menstrual cycle's natural termination.

What is Perimenopause?

The term "perimenopause," which translates literally as "around the menopause," describes the period of transition when menstrual periods start to irregularize. One month you can have a lengthy or heavy menstrual cycle and then miss a cycle the following. It usually begins 4–10 years before menopause in your early to mid-40s, and is frequently indicated by the physical signs of menopause.

Menopause occurs at an average age of 51. Menopause can be a period of immense relief, despite the fact that many women fear it. Hormonal headaches, painful or heavy periods, and PMS symptoms are all relieved by menopause. The days of worrying over which form of birth control to use are over! Menopause is a normal life change for women, and it can be viewed as a new beginning.

The ovaries' erratic production of hormones is what causes the symptoms. Many women experience sporadic symptoms up to ten years before the end of their menstrual cycle.

Menstrual abnormalities, nocturnal sweats, flushing, and sleeplessness are common early signs of menopause.
Women may also experience changes in libido, weight gain, moodiness, and dry vagina.

Concentration problems during menopause are sometimes referred to as "brain fog."

There have also been reports of skin changes, thinning hair, and abdominal bloating.
Every woman has a unique menopausal experience. Some ladies have absolutely no symptoms at all. Usually self-limiting, the symptoms endure between two and three years. Obviously, there are always going to be exceptions; some women claim to have hot flashes far into their seventies. The main point is that these symptoms are temporary.

As women age, this significant shift is unavoidable, and the majority view it as the end of the world. However, despite the fact that you will probably have some symptoms, menopause doesn't have to be as terrible as most women believe it to be.
In actuality, you may navigate menopause with ease and little difficulty if you have the appropriate knowledge and strategies under your belt. Nutrition is a key component in the management of menopause symptoms.

All the components and functions of your body, including the menopausal transition, are greatly influenced by nutrition. By maintaining good

digestion, balancing your nutrient levels, and
ensuring your body has enough antioxidants,
electrolytes, vitamins, minerals, and other
nutrients to function properly, your diet may
help reduce symptoms. Maintaining a nutritious
diet might also aid in controlling any weight
gain.

Furthermore, maintaining a tight eye on your
diet throughout menopause may lower your
chance of contracting a number of conditions
that frequently surface in midlife, including high
blood pressure, type 2 diabetes, high
cholesterol, heart disease, and more. Eating a
nutritious diet also boosts your confidence and
improves your overall mood.

Chapter One

Nutritional needs during menopause

It goes without saying that eating a balanced diet is crucial at every stage of life, but it is a fact that a woman's body undergoes several changes throughout the perimenopause! Oestrogen levels drop, and many women experience alterations in blood pressure and cholesterol levels. This could raise the chance of heart disease.

Furthermore, as calcium is removed from bones, the risk of osteoporosis increases. Regretfully, there's more. Among the symptoms include weight gain, joint pain, hot flashes, nocturnal sweats, irritability, and impaired focus. The decrease in oestrogen levels is the primary cause of all of these symptoms. And so, how do we assist ourselves?

There are several nutrients that we might prioritize to positively influence outcomes while addressing these metabolic problems. These are the principal ones:

Fiber

Research indicates that the bacterial composition of the gut microbiome is changed by the hormonal changes that occur during the menopause transition. This change has a wide range of potential effects on the body, including the heart, stomach, metabolism, and even brain function. In addition to helping to lower cholesterol and improve satiety, fiber is vital for maintaining a healthy gut and blood sugar levels. Even some types of fiber can serve as prebiotics, or nourishment, for the beneficial bacteria in our guts that are part of our biome.

Protein

In terms of satiety and blood sugar control, protein performs many of the same functions as fiber. However, protein also specifically aids in the maintenance of women's functioning. When muscle naturally decreases and doesn't have the same level of support from estrogen for building new muscle,, protein helps maintain and increase muscle mass.

Omega-3 Fatty Acids

Omega-3 fatty acids are an excellent supplement to any diet when it comes to treating the heart health issues connected with menopause. Their capacity to favorably affect triglyceride and cholesterol levels is mostly responsible for this. Foods rich in these beneficial fats also contribute to good weight maintenance by increasing satiety.

Phytoestrogens

Foods high in phytoestrogens are one way we can make up for the estrogen lost during menopause. Plant substances known as phytoestrogens function remarkably similarly to the body's natural oestrogen. This may lessen the intensity and occurrence of some menopausal symptoms, particularly hot flashes.

Water

As estrogen levels drop throughout menopause, staying hydrated becomes even more crucial. Estrogen also contributes to the body's ability to retain water in a positive way. Maintaining enough hydration throughout menopause can benefit the health of your stomach, skin, brain, and joints—preventing constipation, achy joints, and mental fog.

Top Vitamins for Menopause

The following vitamins can aid in symptom relief during your menopause journey. Let's examine them:

Vitamin D

It is essential for reducing hot flashes and preserving bone health. It supports strong bones throughout menopause and aids in regulating the absorption of calcium.

Vitamin B complex

It is an excellent source of nutrients that elevate mood and increase energy. It also decreases irritation and enhances general energy.

Vitamin E

It is well known that vitamin E reduces hot flashes and promotes heart health. This naturally occurring antioxidant may lessen menopausal symptoms.

Magnesium and Calcium

Healthy bones and restful sleep depend on these. When combined, these minerals help with bone health and relaxation.

Vitamin C

It reduces stress and strengthens the immune system. also gives your immune system the assistance it needs throughout menopause.

Vitamin K

It is essential for healthy bones and blood coagulation. It functions in concert with vitamin D to support bone density and reduce the incidence of fractures.

Vitamin A

Vitamin A supports healthy skin and mucous membranes. One common symptom of menopause is decreased vaginal dryness, which is helped by it.

Vitamin B6

This vitamin helps control mood and lessens the typical menopausal symptoms of depression and anxiety.

Vitamin B12

Lessens fatigue and improves overall wellbeing by supporting the maintenance of healthy neurons and energy levels.

Vitamin B5 (Pantothenic acid)

Helps regulate stress levels and the health of the adrenal glands throughout menopause.

Vitamin B3 (Niacin)

This is a type of Vitamin B that promotes good skin and cholesterol levels.

You may naturally reduce the symptoms of menopause by consuming these essential vitamins and nutrients, which will enable you to go through this phase more easily and comfortably.

Chapter Two

Foods to include in the Menopause diet

Protein:

Include protein at every meal and snack if you can. It's not only vital to have a wide variety of proteins, but they also help you feel satiated for longer. Consider including at least one serving of oily fish (salmon, trout, fresh tuna, or mackerel) in your diet each week when selecting protein-rich foods. Select lean meat pieces and don't cook them with an excessive amount of fat.

Like pulses (beans, peas, and lentils), eggs are a fantastic and adaptable food.

As with tofu or Quorn, nuts can be incorporated to a wide range of recipes, such as stir-fries or salads.

Fatty fish:

Numerous studies have connected enhanced mood and cognitive performance to the heart-healthy omega-3 fatty acids found in fish. Additionally, omega-3 fatty acids can aid in controlling blood pressure. Hot flashes may be easier to manage with normal blood pressure. One of the few food sources of vitamin D, an essential component for bone health and mood, is fatty fish like salmon.

Carbohydrates:

Many individuals find carbohydrates to be puzzling and perceive them as the enemy. While some carbohydrates are beneficial, such as those found in sugary cakes and biscuits, everyone should restrict their intake of them. There are some "good" carbohydrates, though. These include potatoes, pasta, cereals, and grains; we need them for energy and fiber. Speaking of fiber, try to eat potatoes with their skin on and, whenever possible, choose whole grain pasta and cereal.

Dairy and substitutes:

Women frequently experience a decrease in strength throughout menopause, so it's important to make sure you're getting the nutrients your bones need to be healthy and preserve their density. Calcium and vitamin D are the two important elements for healthy bones. To guarantee that their levels stay healthy, women should take a vitamin D supplement every day (400 IU or 10 micrograms advised).

A simple three servings of dairy every day can help us maintain our calcium levels in various ways. This could be 200ml of milk, 25g of cheese, yoghurt, or even a milk-based dish like rice pudding. Many alternatives, including soy, nut, oat, rice, and yoghurt milks, are available for people who prefer to forgo dairy. Just make sure you add calcium to fortify them.

Fruits and vegetables:

Diversity is important in this case; if you can, try to consume a rainbow of hues that represent various vitamins and minerals. Everyone knows that you should only have five a day, but you can certainly have a few more! Not only do fresh fruits and vegetables qualify, but canned or frozen goods also do. These are often less costly!

Beverages:

In addition to water, keep in mind that smoothies, fruit juice, and alcohol do not count towards your daily fluid consumption. Though tea, coffee, and herbal variations do work, try limiting your daily consumption to one or two cups or opting for decaf kinds if you experience hot flashes or have trouble falling asleep.

Other foods or supplements:

As mentioned above, taking a daily vitamin D supplement is advised. If you find it difficult to eat oily fish, you might also want to think about taking omega 3 fish oil supplements. Just be careful to purchase high-quality goods.

Some women have reported that the frequency and intensity of hot flashes can be reduced by using plant oestrogens, also referred to as phytoestrogens. Women in their 40s have shown to have the best outcomes. Over the course of two to three months, 2-3 portions of plant-based, estrogen-rich food, such as soya, would need to be ingested daily in order to have the optimum outcomes.

Snacks:

Everyone experiences occasional hunger between meals, but avoid grabbing high-fat, high-sugar snacks as these may exacerbate your symptoms! Rather, focus your snack on fruit and protein or carbs and protein. A tiny matchbox piece of cheese with two oatcakes, sliced apple with peanut butter, dried fruit with unsalted almonds, or a small bread roll with a banana are a few healthy alternatives.

Healthy Foods to consume during Menopause

Yogurt

Yogurt is a fantastic choice for menopausal women since it is high in probiotics and protein that builds muscle. Probiotics are beneficial bacteria that contribute to the gut microbiome's population growth. It's also loaded with calcium, which strengthens bones. In fact, a study on postmenopausal women revealed a significant correlation between dairy consumption and bone strength. Alternative yogurts can also be helpful if you don't eat dairy for whatever reason (though the amount of protein, calcium, and probiotics may vary depending on the brand).

Salmon:

If you're going through menopause, there are a ton of reasons to appreciate salmon. Its protein, omega-3 fatty acids, and vitamin D content are responsible for this. Moreover, salmon has a lot of tryptophan, an amino acid that promotes restful sleep. There are many delectable ways to enjoy this beloved pink fish, whether it's sautéed with lemon and garlic or beautifully arranged over capers, red onion, cream cheese, and a whole wheat bagel.

Berries:

Any berry will work wonders for a menopausal care regimen, whether you choose raspberries, strawberries, blueberries, blackberries, goji berries, or cranberries. These berries include lots of heart-healthy fiber, refreshing water, and phytoestrogens. They'll also provide an abundance of magnesium, potassium, and vitamin K for healthy bones.

Grapes:

Rich in water, fiber, copper, vitamin K, and the powerful anti-inflammatory compound resveratrol, grapes are also a fantastic source of phytoestrogens. A small randomized control trial found that grape seed extract helped women suffering menopause symptoms by lowering blood pressure and improving muscle composition.

Legumes:

When it comes to plant-based protein sources, legumes are hard to match. Any type of legume—chickpeas, lentils, soy beans, black beans, or whatever else you can think of—will provide a great supply of fiber and protein that builds muscle. Packed with phytoestrogens, chickpeas and soy products like edamame and tofu are especially fantastic complements.

Kale:

One excellent leafy green to utilize for managing menopause symptoms is kale. Its high fiber, water, calcium, vitamin K, and manganese levels are responsible for this. Together, these nutrients promote gut and bone health in addition to hydration.

Flaxseeds:

Hemp and chia seeds are great for women going through menopause, but flaxseeds may be the best option. Its remarkable concentrations of fiber, protein, omega-3 fatty acids, and phytoestrogens are the reason for this. But before you eat them, grind your flaxseeds to release their nutrients and other valuable properties.

Green Tea:

Green tea is a nutritious drink to have throughout the menopausal periods. It's an excellent source of phytoestrogen and other anti-inflammatory plant chemicals. Compared to coffee and black teas, it has less caffeine, which helps promote better sleep, proper hydration, and consistent energy levels throughout the day.

Oats:

Oats are particularly great for a healthy menopause diet, mainly because of their high soluble fiber content. All whole grains are good for this. This type of fiber aids in the removal of cholesterol from the body by binding to it in the small intestine. It stabilizes blood sugar and boosts satiety while acting as a prebiotic for our gut bacteria.

Bone broth:

Glycine and proline are two amino acids found in bone broth. Healthy serotonin levels, which promote deeper, more peaceful sleep—something that can be compromised during menopause—are supported by glycine. Not only does this flavorful broth typically have high levels of potassium, magnesium, and phosphorus, but it also helps maintain bone density. Not to mention the ample amount of hydration that this liquid gold offers.

Foods to avoid during Menopause

Limiting items that can worsen symptoms is just as important during menopause as focusing on getting the nutrition you need. Here are some of the offenders to be wary of:

Spicy foods:

Unsurprisingly, eating spicy food might exacerbate hot flashes. Eat less spicy foods like cayenne, jalapenos, and hot peppers if you have high blood pressure or if you tend to feel hot all the time.

Alcohol:

It's unlikely that a few glasses of wine per week will have an impact on your symptoms. However, consuming more than one drink each day (12 ounces of beer, 5 ounces of wine, or 1.5 ounces of spirits are all considered drinks) may have a negative impact on your health and wellbeing. Alcohol disrupts sleep, and it can make anxiety, melancholy, and hot flashes worse. You can gain weight as well if your lower inhibitions push you to the kitchen.

Fatty foods:

Try limiting your consumption of foods high in fat, unless they're nuts or fatty seafood. Eat less processed food, quick food, fried food, and cookies, cakes, and snacks.

Chapter Three

Hydration Importance

When considering dietary modifications during menopause, it is easy to lose sight of the importance of fluids in favor of food. But they are just as vital to our well-being as the nutrients we get from the food we eat.

Why is it important to stay hydrated?

It's common knowledge that staying hydrated is important, and for good reason. Body cells are mostly made of fluids. These liquids support a variety of body functions, many of which are essential to our existence. As an illustration, fluids:
- Transport oxygen and nutrients throughout the circulatory system.
- Assist the kidneys in eliminating waste from the body through urine
- Joint lubrication
- Wet the lips, nose, and eyes.
- Aid in controlling body temperature.

Signs of Dehydration:

If the body is losing more fluids than it is taking in, dehydration may result. This is usually the result of consuming insufficient amounts of water. We all know that prolonged dehydration can result in kidney stones, constipation, and increased frequency of UTIs, therefore it's best to prevent it.
Among the most typical transient signs of dehydration are:

- Feeling thirsty
- Dizziness
- Tongue, lips, and mouth feeling dry
- Feeling tired
- Headaches
- Sporadic urination
- Urine smells strongly of dark yellow

How much water should you drink to relieve menopausal symptoms and dehydration?

Divide your body weight in half to determine how much fluids you should drink each day, That equates to 60 ounces a day for a 120-pound person. Your daily urination frequency will undoubtedly change if you drink more water and to make up for the extra water lost, you need even more if you experience hot flashes and nocturnal sweats. Drinking enough water will also help you feel less fatigued and dizzy throughout the menopause.

Two thirds of the 60 ounces should be water. "Other" items, including juice, tea, or coffee, can make up the remaining third.

According to a 2013 research, not nearly half of Americans drank enough water. The study also found that our attitudes toward water deteriorate with age. As we age, our thirst perception decreases, so if you're worried you're not drinking enough, it might be time to monitor your consumption.

Avoiding dehydration during Menopause

In the same way that a withered flower reemerges after a refreshing downpour, a well hydrated human organism flourishes. We all know that being hydrated is crucial for general health and wellbeing, but as we approach menopause, the importance of this habit increases.

Not only may drinking enough water ease some of the discomfort related to menopause, but drinking too little water might potentially induce or worsen some menopause symptoms. Let's examine the importance of staying hydrated during menopause and some practical strategies for doing so.

Hydration can help reduce some menopause symptoms

Important biological processes including temperature regulation, joint lubrication and cushioning, and waste elimination are all made possible by water, which is necessary for life.

In actuality, water makes about 60% of the human body on average; however, following menopause, this number may decrease to 55% for women.

Your level of hydration becomes more important during menopause because, as previously discussed, it can either help with or make some menopause symptoms worse.

Body water content decreases with age and menopause, partly because of decreased estrogen levels. It's crucial to stay hydrated at any age. It's especially beneficial for people coping with menopausal hot flashes and night sweats, which can result in excessive sweating and dehydration.

The following are a few symptoms that drinking enough water may assist with:

Bladder Irritation

Because of increased vaginal dryness or skin thinning brought on by estrogen loss, some menopausal women may have pain when they urinate. It has been demonstrated that drinking lots of water can help reduce some of this discomfort and agony in the urine. Increasing the amount of fluid consumed helps to dilute the urine and may also prevent the growth of some germs that could irritate and hurt the bladder. Maintaining adequate hydration helps to avoid highly concentrated pee and may also alleviate associated bladder irritation. Furthermore, drinking enough water helps to flush the urinary tract, which may assist to prevent infections.

Dry Skin

Women may notice dry, itchy skin after menopause because estrogen increases the development of collagen and oils that keep skin firm and moisturised. Dryness may also result from the skin's decreased capacity to hold onto water during the menopause. Since water makes up the majority of our body's cells and tissues, drinking enough water can help moisturize your skin from the inside out. Even during menopause, drinking enough water can encourage the creation of collagen.

Headaches

Migraines and other types of headaches are frequently linked to changes in hormone levels that occur after menopause. Drinking water may help reduce headaches because underlying dehydration might exacerbate them. Dehydration brought on by menopausal heat flashes has also been linked to headaches. Staying hydrated is even more crucial during a hot flash since you can lose more water owing to increased sweat.

Dehydration can worsen Some menopause symptoms

While dehydration might exacerbate many menopausal symptoms, drinking enough of water can assist with others. Among the menopausal symptoms that dehydration might make worse are:

Brain fog

A just 1% dehydration is sufficient to cause a 5% decline in cognitive abilities. If a woman has menopausal brain fog, dehydration may exacerbate her symptoms. Research has indicated a connection between brain function and dehydration, which can have deleterious effects on executive functions, attention span, and critical motor skills.

Fatigue

One of the symptoms that many menopausal women encounter is fatigue. Poor sleep brought on by anything from sleeplessness to night sweats could be the problem. However, exhaustion can also occur during the day and is occasionally brought on by menopausal hormone swings. Since that a healthy body and mind depend on water, dehydration itself may be the cause. Whatever the cause, the next time you're feeling down, take stock of yourself. One of the first things you should do to fight weariness is to make sure you're getting enough water.

Aching joints

Some women may have joint pain and swelling during menopause when their levels of estrogen, which lowers inflammation, fall. Uric acid accumulation in the joints brought on by dehydration can exacerbate joint discomfort.

How to drink enough water during menopause

I'm sure you've heard the recommendation to have eight glasses of water each day. For women going through menopause, the conventional eight glasses per day norm still holds true. The best water is plain, with or without electrolytes.

Aside from this general guideline, there are other circumstances in which you might need to consume more fluids:

Exercise

It's a good idea to try to replace the fluids your body loses via sweat by drinking water prior to, during, and after exercise. Menopause makes it even more crucial to maintain an active lifestyle because studies have shown that it can improve mood, improve sleep quality, and even lower your chance of developing certain diseases like heart disease. To prevent dehydration, keep active but also maintain your fluid intake.

Hot Weather

Similar to physical activity, excessive perspiration on hot days can result in fluid loss, necessitating increased hydration. Menopausal hot flashes might also be more common in certain women during the scorching summer months. In order to control your skin temperature and prevent a hot flash, if you plan to go outside during the summer, think about carrying a fan or a water bottle with you.

Illness or Other Health Concerns

Extra water may be needed by your body if you've been sick. Water is essential for the proper operation of all body cells, including immune system cells. Both a fever and the normal GI symptoms of vomiting and diarrhea result in increased sweating and water loss. Water replenishment is vitally necessary. Generally speaking, the color of your pee is a good indicator of your state of hydration. You're probably properly hydrated if your pee is clear and pale yellow; if it's black and concentrated, you might need to drink extra water.

Which Fluids Are the Greatest for Hydration?

For the best possible hydration, nothing beats water, but you don't need to down many glasses to meet your needs. Another way to consume water is through the consumption of fruits and vegetables that are high in water content. Watermelon gets its name from its 92% water content, whereas cantaloupe and strawberries have about 90% water content. Lettuce and cucumbers are high in hydration as well.

Whether it's from activity, warm weather, or menopausal hot flashes, you may want to think about drinking something like coconut water or a sports drink that helps replenish electrolytes if you've been perspiring. Research indicates that replenishing lost electrolytes and water is necessary for achieving rehydration following perspiration.

Which Beverages Need to be Avoided?

Are there certain drinks that women should stay away from during menopause in order to stay hydrated? Fortunately, drinking coffee and other caffeinated beverages in moderation is unlikely to cause dehydration. Due to its diuretic properties, caffeine may make you need to urinate more frequently. However, studies show that caffeine wouldn't have diuretic effect until you drank more than five cups of brewed coffee a day.

On the other hand, alcohol should be used in moderation or avoided because it has stronger diuretic effects and can quickly cause dehydration. Additionally, the effects of alcohol on the body may vary between the perimenopause and menopause. Drinking in excess of moderation—roughly seven drinks per week—can cause problems and possibly exacerbate menopausal symptoms, according to the North American Menopause Society (NAMS).

Chapter Four

Menopause diet meal plan

What is a Menopause diet plan?
A menopause diet plan is a manner of eating that can enhance general health and assist in managing menopausal symptoms. Eating an abundance of unprocessed foods, such as fruits, vegetables, whole grains, lean protein, and healthy fats, is the foundation of this approach.

Menopausal weight loss:

Five unexpected foods to stay away from

If you're attempting to shed pounds after menopause, you might want to limit or stay away from these five unexpected foods:

Fruit Juice:

Although fruit juice is frequently promoted as a healthful beverage, it can be heavy in calories and sugar. For instance, a cup of orange juice has roughly 22 grams of sugar and 110 calories. Eating whole fruits is preferable than drinking fruit juice because the fiber in whole fruits helps to slow down the bloodstream's absorption of sugar.

Yogurt parfaits:

Although yogurt parfaits are sometimes promoted as a nutritious breakfast choice, they can be heavy in calories and sugar. Granola, yogurt, and fruit combined in a parfait can have more than 400 calories and 50 grams of sugar in it. It's better to make your yogurt parfait at home with tiny amounts of granola and basic, fresh fruit.

Dried Fruit:

Another seemingly healthful food that may be heavy in sugar is dried fruit. For instance, 210 calories and 50 grams of sugar are found in one cup of dried cranberries. When selecting dried fruit, it's crucial to carefully read the nutrition label and choose for types that are high in fiber and low in sugar.

Whole-wheat bread:

Although whole-wheat bread is frequently regarded as a better option than white bread, it can still contain a lot of sugar and calories. A single piece of whole-wheat bread may have 15 grams of sugar and 70 calories. Selecting whole-wheat bread that has a high fiber content and little added sugar is crucial.

Energy drinks:

Energy drinks might be detrimental to your health despite their common claims to increase energy and enhance performance. Energy drinks are heavy in sugar, artificial chemicals, and caffeine. They might also lead to other health problems, like dehydration.

During menopause, maintaining weight control and supporting general health require a balanced diet.

Ideal diet plan for weight loss during Menopause

The ideal food plan for weight loss during menopause is tailored to your individual needs and tastes. Nonetheless, throughout this period, you can minimize belly fat and lose weight by following some fundamental guidelines.

Consume lots of protein:

Consuming protein can help you cut calories since it keeps you feeling full and content. Lean meat, chicken, fish, beans, lentils, and tofu are all excellent sources of protein. Add some good fats to your diet: Good fats may aid in weight loss and in the reduction of inflammation. Nuts, seeds, avocados, and olive oil are good sources of good fats.

Consume a lot of fiber:

In addition to keeping you full and content, fiber can assist lose abdominal fat. Whole grains, beans, lentils, vegetables, and fruits are all excellent providers of dietary fiber.

Limit sugar-filled beverages, processed foods, and harmful fats:

Sugar-filled beverages, processed foods, and unhealthy fats are low in nutrients and heavy in calories. likewise, they may be a factor in gaining weight and belly fat.

Ensure you are getting enough water:

Drinking enough water is beneficial to your general health and can aid in weight loss.

Hormonal changes associated with menopause might make weight control more difficult, but with the correct strategy, it is still feasible to reach and maintain a healthy weight.

The following are some essential guidelines for a menopause weight loss diet that work:

A balanced diet

Make a point of eating a varied range of foods
from all the food groups, such as fruits,
vegetables, whole grains, lean meats, and
healthy fats, as part of a balanced diet. This
helps suppress appetite and supplies vital
nutrients.

Portion control:

Pay attention to portion proportions to prevent
eating too much. Use smaller portions and be
mindful of your body's signals of fullness and
hunger.

Select Whole Foods:

Complete, unprocessed foods are preferable to
heavily processed ones. In general, whole
foods are healthier and more full.
Lean Protein: Include foods high in protein,
such as fish, poultry, tofu, beans, and lentils
throughout your meals. During menopause,
muscular mass can decrease; protein helps to
retain it.
Good Fats: Add foods like avocados, almonds,
seeds, and olive oil to your diet as sources of

good fats. These fats can improve your general health and make you feel pleased.

Stress Management:

Use ways to reduce stress such as yoga, meditation, or deep breathing. Excessive stress levels have been linked to weight growth.

Weekly meal plan for weight loss during Menopause

This is a sample of a Menopause weight loss weekly meal plan:

Day 1

Breakfast:

- Nuts and berries in oatmeal

Lunch:

- Quinoa, veggies, and grilled fish or chicken in a salad.

Dinner:

- Roasted vegetables served with salmon.

Day 2

Breakfast:

- Granola and fruit paired with yogurt

Lunch:

- Pairing whole-wheat bread with lentil soup

Dinner:

- Stir-fried chicken over brown rice

Day 3

Breakfast:

- Avocado with whole-wheat bread with eggs

Lunch:

- A whole-wheat baguette topped with a veggie burger and sweet potato fries

Dinner:

- Meatballs with tomato sauce over lentil pasta

Day 4

Breakfast:

- Smoothie including protein powder, yogurt, and fruit

Lunch:

- Leftovers from the meal

Dinner:

- Lunch leftovers

Day 5

Breakfast:

- Pancakes made with whole wheat, berries, and yogurt

Lunch:

- Vegetables and tuna salad sandwich on whole-wheat bread

Dinner:

- Whole-wheat bread paired with vegetarian chili

Day 6

Breakfast:

- Berries and chia seeds for overnight oats

Lunch:

- Quinoa bowl with chickpeas and roasted veggies

Dinner:

- Sweet potato fries served with salmon patties

Day 7

Breakfast:

- Hard-boiled eggs, avocado, and whole-wheat bread

Lunch:

- Quinoa, veggies, and grilled tofu in a salad

Dinner:

- Roasted veggies and chicken breast

This meal plan is low in processed foods, sugar-filled beverages, and bad fats and high in protein, fiber, and healthy fats. It's also critical to remember that this meal plan is merely a sample. It can be modified to suit your unique requirements and tastes.

Perimenopause diet plan to lose weight

The same guidelines that apply to a menopause diet plan should also apply to perimenopause diet plans for weight loss, with a few modification.

Here are some particular pointers for formulating a weight-loss diet plan during the perimenopause:

Consume lots of protein:

You can consume less calories when you consume protein since it keeps you feeling full and content. Lean meat, chicken, fish, beans, lentils, and tofu are all excellent sources of protein.

Select complex carbs rather than simple ones:

Because complex carbs breakdown more slowly than simple ones, they can help control blood sugar levels and reduce cravings. Whole fruits, vegetables, and grains are good sources of complex carbs.

Minimize sugar-filled drinks:

Sugar-filled drinks have little nutritional benefit and are heavy in calories. Water, unsweetened tea, or coffee are better options.

Include more good fats in your diet:

Good fats have anti-inflammatory and satiety properties. Nuts, seeds, Avocados, and Olive oil are all excellent sources of good fats.

This is a sample of a weight-loss meal plan for a perimenopause diet:

Breakfast:

- Oatmeal mixed with nuts and fruit.

- Granola and fruit with yogurt.

- Avocados with whole-wheat bread with eggs

Lunch:

- Salad paired with fish or grilled chicken.

- Lentil soup

- Wrap made of whole wheat, hummus, and veggies.

Dinner

- Roasted veggies and salmon.

- Stir-fried quinoa with tofu.

- Meatballs with tomato sauce over lentil pasta

Snacks:

- Yogurt, fruits, veggies, nuts, and seeds.

Additionally, you might try include a few of the following tips in your diet:

Consume regular meals and snacks:

This will lessen cravings and help you maintain stable blood sugar levels.

Ensure you are getting enough water:

Reducing hunger and increasing metabolism are two benefits of being hydrated.

Engage in regular exercise:

Exercise can aid in weight loss and is beneficial to general health. On most days of the week, try to engage in moderate-intense activity for at least half an hour.

In summary

A diet that is well-balanced and customized to meet personal preferences and needs is essential for women going through menopause or perimenopause.

Lean proteins, good fats, lots of fiber, and whole, unprocessed foods should all be included in this diet, with a restriction on processed and sugary foods.

In addition to food choices, consistent exercise, stress reduction, and enough hydration all play important roles in managing weight throughout this period of life.

It's critical to keep in mind that each person is different, therefore seeking individualized advice from a medical professional or certified dietitian is advised for successful and long-lasting weight loss during menopause.

Chapter Five

Supplements for Menopausal women

Hormone replacement therapy (HRT) has been the main treatment for menopausal symptoms, but many women are unable to use it or do not want to because of the health hazards.
More than 50% of women are thought to treat their problems using complementary and alternative medicine, and 60% of them believe these non-traditional approaches are a good way to get relief. These include holistic methods (acupuncture, reflexology, and homeopathy), mind-body activities (yoga, meditation, and aromatherapy), and dietary supplements (vitamins, herbs, and minerals).

The following supplements may provide relief from menopausal symptoms.

Melatonin

The pineal gland naturally produces melatonin, a hormone that aids in controlling sleep-wake cycles. Taking melatonin may aid with sleep since it decreases with age and sleeplessness is a frequent menopause symptom.
Melatonin not only promotes sleep, but a tiny study demonstrated that women taking 3 mg of the hormone improved in physical symptoms related to the perimenopause when compared to controls. The study also discovered that supplementing with melatonin may help stop bone loss, although additional investigation is required.

Furthermore, a study that supplemented perimenopausal women with 3 mg of melatonin for six months reported significant benefits in menopause-related sadness and thyroid function.

Vitamin D and calcium

Bone health may suffer as a result of
perimenopause-related estrogen decline. It's
critical to have enough calcium and vitamin D
in particular, as well as other vitamins and
minerals, to maintain healthy bones.
For women aged 18 to 50, the recommended
daily allowance (RDA) for calcium is 1,000 mg.
The RDA is increased to 1,200 mg after age
50. You can consume foods high in calcium or
take supplements. Green leafy vegetables,
dairy and soy products, fish (especially
sardines) with bones, and fortified beverages
are good sources of calcium.
Getting enough vitamin D is crucial to support
calcium absorption, regardless of whether you
get your calcium from food or supplements.

Vitamin D is naturally found in sunlight, but
many people don't get enough of it, particularly
those who live in colder climates or have dark
skin. While the US Institute of Medicine
suggests consuming 400–800 IU on average
per day, some research suggests exceeding
this amount to reach the safe top range of
1000–4000 IU.

The following other minerals are crucial for healthy bones: magnesium, potassium, vitamin K, and vitamin C. Eat a lot of plant foods (particularly fruits, vegetables, and legumes) to ensure you receive enough. To make sure you're meeting all of your nutritional needs, you might also want to take a multivitamin that is appropriate for your age and gender. Additionally, studies have indicated that postmenopausal women may have higher bone mineral density if they take 5g of collagen peptides daily.

Another excellent strategy to boost muscle mass and bone density—both of which tend to decline as estrogen levels drop—is through exercise. Eat enough protein to support your muscle mass even more. For women over 50, the recommended daily allowance (RDA) for protein is higher than for younger women: 1 to 1.5 grams per kilogram of body weight (1 kilogram = 2.2 pounds). 20–25 grams should be consumed at each meal.

Omega 3's

Recent studies have demonstrated that omega-3 fatty acids can lessen the psychological discomfort and depressed symptoms that menopausal and perimenopausal women frequently experience. In addition to lowering joint pain, taking a high-quality Omega-3 supplement helps shield women's hearts and bones.

Magnesium

Magnesium relieves anxiety and sleep problems associated with menopausal and perimenopausal hormone abnormalities. In addition, magnesium helps prevent osteoporosis, lower blood pressure, strengthen the heart, and ease constipation—especially if you take magnesium glycinate. Since the majority of women's diets are deficient in magnesium, taking a magnesium supplement is frequently essential for symptom relief.

Phytoestrogens

"Phytoestrogens," which are abundant in fruits and vegetables, are especially helpful for women experiencing hot flashes and other menopausal symptoms. Isoflavones and lignans are two examples of phytoestrogens; these substances gently assist your body in readjusting the hormonal balance at the cellular level.

Because they contain isoflavones, soy beans and meals prepared from them, such as tofu, are rich in phytoestrogens. Another excellent option is flax seeds due to their high lignan content. Every day, grind up one to three teaspoons of flax seeds and use them into smoothies, salads, and soups. Additionally, a variety of seeds, nuts, and legumes as well as celery, fennel, parsley, garlic, and onions contain phytoestrogens.

Herbal remedies for Menopause .

For generations, women have used traditional herbal medicines to address a wide range of menopausal symptoms, including PMS, anxiety, sadness, and insomnia. The most well-liked herbs for boosting sleep and lowering anxiety include chamomile, passionflower, lavender, and valerian.

Herbs and other plants can be kinder to the body than medications, assisting in the healing process. They are ingested as teas, tinctures, or tablets. Some can be added to dishes like stews, soups, and smoothies. Remember that herbal medicine can be potent, so it's a good idea to discuss your medications with your doctor. Integrative and complementary medicine is also widely used by physicians.

These additional herbs might be useful in treating menopausal symptoms.

Black Cohosh

Black cohosh is one of the most well-liked and researched herbs for menopausal symptoms. The roots of this plant, which were first employed by Native Americans and were sometimes referred to as "bugbane" since they were used as an insect repellant, are gathered in the Fall and can be used either fresh or dried for medical purposes. Chemicals in the plant have an impact on the neurological and immunological systems, and they may also help regulate estrogen.

St. John's Wort

For generations, people have utilized the wild plant St. John's wort to improve their mental well-being. It is available for purchase as a dietary supplement and is prescribed for depression in Europe.
Studies examining the impact of taking three times daily doses of St. John's wort for a full year discovered that the herbal treatment significantly reduced the psychological and psychosomatic symptoms experienced by women who were experiencing menopausal

symptoms. Another study indicated that women treated with St. John's wort had much higher quality of life related to the menopause and experienced less sleep problems than controls. The ladies using St. John's wort also showed a decrease in hot flashes.

Wild yam

Wild yam is a tuber that has been used for millennia in traditional Chinese medicine to alleviate menopausal symptoms. It is well-known as a natural substitute for estrogen therapy. It is frequently added to creams and has a substance called diosgenin that may be converted into several steroids, including estrogen, in a lab. Despite the fact that wild yam does not seem to produce estrogen in the body, the plant might contain other substances that do.
A randomized clinical experiment including 50 women who took 12 mg of purple yam twice a day revealed significant reductions in menopausal symptoms (mainly psychological) compared to controls, however more research is required to confirm its efficacy.

Dong Quai

Dong quai, a member of the carrot and celery family and essential component of Chinese herbal medicine, is widely used to boost immunity and reduce inflammation. It's called "female ginseng" a lot. It is used to treat menopause and menstrual cramps as well as to regulate a woman's hormones.

Maca

Maca is a cruciferous vegetable that is indigenous to the Andes Mountains of Peru. It belongs to the mustard family. In traditional medicine, the root is said to boost libido and fertility. It is frequently used in Peruvian cookery and has a rich, earthy flavor. Rich in iron, copper, and vitamin C, it can also be taken as a supplement and added to meals or smoothies as a powder.

In Summary

It is crucial to realize that every woman has a unique menopausal experience. While some get by easily, others find it difficult. Whatever

you are going through, take it easy and be kind
on yourself, and prioritize taking care of
yourself.

Consult your pharmacist or doctor if you use
any supplements. Remember that:

Every supplements have potential side effects.
Herbs and supplements may interact with
some of the medications you take. They could
increase or decrease the effects of medication.
Alternatively, the interaction can result in more
issues.
Allergies can occur from certain herbs.

Chapter Six

Physical activity and its impacts

Women are believed to benefit greatly from physical activity both during and after menopause since living a healthy lifestyle can lower your risk of disease and maintain a healthy heart.

Advantages of exercise

There are several advantages in engaging in regular physical activity both before and after menopause. These include:

- Preventing weight gain, as women going through menopause often lose muscle mass and develop stomach fat.

- Reduce the incidence of fractures and osteoporosis by strengthening bones and slowing down bone loss.

- Lower your chance of developing illnesses like Type 2 Diabetes, which is a result of rapid weight gain.

Activities that can be beneficial

For women going through menopause, aerobic activity and strength training are the two main forms of exercise that are advised. Exercise that works your big muscle groups and raises your heart rate is called aerobic exercise. Aerobic exercise comes in various forms.

Walking: When done at a fast speed, walking is the most basic type of low-impact aerobic exercise and burns calories.

Swimming is an additional low-impact cardiovascular exercise that is less taxing on the joints than other exercises like running.

Dancing is a fantastic low-impact aerobic exercise that burns calories and can be a lot of fun.

You should begin with a mild cardio exercise, such as walking, swimming, dancing, running, or riding a bike, especially if you haven't worked out on a regular basis for some time. As you feel yourself getting fitter, progressively increase the duration and intensity of your activity.

Because strength training is an excellent method of burning calories, building muscle, and losing body fat, it is also advised for women going through and beyond menopause. Hand-held weights, resistance training, and weight machines are examples of strength training methods. Because osteoporosis is more likely to occur as estrogen levels fall throughout menopause, this kind of activity is very crucial for strengthening bones.

When doing strength training, select a weight or resistance level that causes your muscles to become fatigued after around twelve repetitions. Then, when you start to feel stronger, progressively increase that level. Aim for three sessions of strength training per week.

Exercise Tips

If you choose to begin an exercise regimen during or after menopause, bear the following advice in mind:

- Attempt to engage in strong aerobic activity for at least 75 minutes per week, or double that amount if you only engage in moderate aerobic exercise.

- To keep your routine from becoming boring, make sure you set reasonable and doable goals for yourself. You should also update and modify it periodically.

- Make an effort to enjoy your workout routine. Exercise is something you can do anywhere, and tasks around the house and in the garden can also be considered exercise.

- Make sure you begin with mild exercise and work your way up to more strenuous exercises. Always remember to warm up and cool down before and after working out.

Engaging in physical activity is advantageous throughout our entire life. It strengthens our hearts, encourages weight loss, and increases our level of fitness. In addition to its potential to prevent disease, physical activity during and after menopause is thought to be beneficial in lowering menopausal symptoms such stress, anxiety, and depression.

Chapter Seven

Managing weight during Menopause

A woman's natural menopause phase is marked by a number of changes, including weight gain. But do not worry! You can control your weight throughout this period of change if you have the appropriate information and techniques. We'll look at the relationship between menopause and weight gain, how it affects your health, and how to assist your weight management journey with dietary advice, exercise routines, and lifestyle modifications in this book.

Understanding Menopause and weight gain

When a woman enters the menopause, which usually happens in her late 40s or early 50s, she stops having periods. It is associated with a range of physiological and hormonal changes and signifies the end of the reproductive years. Gaining weight is one of the most frequent worries women have at this period. Many women do suffer an increase in weight, especially around the belly, however it is not inevitable. Let's examine the relationship between weight increase and menopause in more detail.

The relationship between Menopause and weight gain

The drop in estrogen levels during menopause is one of the main causes of weight gain. The hormone estrogen, which is generated by the ovaries, aids in controlling body weight by preserving a normal metabolism. It is essential for spreading fat throughout the body and making sure it is stored in the proper locations. But as women get closer to menopause, their estrogen levels start to drop, upsetting this delicate equilibrium.

Your body may accumulate more fat as estrogen levels drop, particularly around the waist. This is because, in comparison to other parts of the body, fat cells in the abdominal region have a higher amount of estrogen receptors. They so tend to gain fat more easily and are more susceptible to hormonal fluctuations. Your total weight may rise as a result of this shift in fat distribution, and your body composition may also alter.

Common causes for weight gain during Menopause

Menopausal weight gain is largely caused by hormonal changes, although they are not the only cause. This phenomena is caused by a number of other causes, making it a complex problem that calls for an all-encompassing strategy to effectively address.

One of the main causes of weight increase during menopause is decreased physical activity. Women tend to become less active as they get older, which causes their metabolism to slow down and their muscular mass to decrease. The body's capacity to burn calories effectively is further diminished by this loss of muscle mass, increasing the likelihood of weight gain.

Genetic predisposition can also affect weight gain after menopause, in addition to physical activity. It's possible that some women are genetically predisposed to gaining weight quickly, particularly during hormonal changes. Although genetics cannot be altered, women can take proactive measures to properly manage their weight by being aware of this inclination.

A significant contributing factor to menopausal weight gain is lifestyle choices. Weight gain can be attributed to poor dietary choices, such as consuming an excessive amount of processed meals and sugary drinks. Menopause weight gain can also be exacerbated by stress, sleep deprivation, and emotional problems that might result in overeating or bad eating habits.

It's critical to remember that weight gain during menopause has practical implications beyond appearance. Being overweight raises the risk of heart disease, diabetes, and joint issues, among other illnesses. Thus, throughout this stage of life, it is imperative to take a holistic approach to weight management.

Women who comprehend the relationship between menopause and weight gain and the elements that contribute to it can create tactics that work effectively for them in maintaining a healthy weight. Regular exercise, a healthy diet, stress reduction methods, and asking for help from medical professionals or support groups are a few examples of these tactics.

Menopausal weight gain's impact on health

Even though it's normal to gain weight during menopause, it's important to understand the possible health hazards linked to weight gain.

Hormonal changes during menopause might cause weight gain, especially around the abdomen. A woman's self-image and general well-being may be impacted by this weight gain, which can be upsetting.

Risks to Physical Health

Being overweight raises the risk of heart disease, high blood pressure, diabetes, and some types of cancer, among other ailments. The buildup of fat around the waist can be especially dangerous because it raises the risk of cardiovascular illnesses.

Moreover, menopausal weight gain may be a factor in joint pain and discomfort. The added weight increases wear and tear on the joints by applying more pressure. This may lead to crippling ailments like osteoarthritis, which lower a person's quality of life.

Issues with Mental Health

Menopause-related weight gain may also have an effect on mental health. A lot of women report feeling less confident in their bodies and less satisfied with them. A negative body image and a feeling of losing control over one's appearance can result from changes in body size and shape.

Furthermore, weight gain during menopause might have emotional effects that go beyond issues with body image. Hormonal changes can be a factor in mood swings, impatience, and a heightened sense of worry or depression. It is imperative that women put their mental health first and get help when they need it.

Techniques for Managing Weight Gain During Menopause

Even though menopausal weight gain might be difficult to regulate, there are methods for keeping a healthy weight:

- Exercise on a regular basis to maintain muscle mass, burn calories, and increase metabolism. Try to integrate cardiovascular, strength, and flexibility training into your daily activities.

- Maintain a well-balanced diet by emphasizing the consumption of foods high in nutrients, such as fruits, vegetables, whole grains, lean meats, and healthy fats. Minimize processed foods and sugary snacks as well as drinks.

- Learn portion control by paying attention to portion sizes and your body's signals of hunger and fullness. Avoid eating past the point of fullness.

- Control your stress: Stress might impede your attempts to lose weight and lead to weight gain. Include stress-reduction methods in your everyday practice, such as mindfulness, meditation, and relaxation exercises.

- Seek expert advice: Speak with a medical practitioner or certified dietitian for individualized guidance and assistance in handling menopausal weight gain.

Women can overcome the difficulties of menopausal weight gain and advance general health and happiness by using a comprehensive strategy that takes into account both physical and emotional well-being.

Chapter Eight

Addressing specific symptoms

Changes in hormone levels during the menopause transition might impact your menstrual cycle and result in symptoms like hot flashes and difficulty sleeping. As you approach menopause, you might have additional symptoms like irregular periods, pain during intercourse, and urinary issues. Discuss your symptoms with your physician or a nurse. Medications and other therapies may be able to reduce your symptoms.

Hot flashes

The most typical menopausal symptom is hot flashes, also known as hot flushes. Hot flashes affect up to three of every four women. When they are still getting their periods, some women start experiencing hot flashes prior to menopause.

An abrupt sensation of heat in the upper torso is known as a hot flash. You might get flushed in the face and neck. You can get red spots on your arms, back, and chest. Along with excessive sweating, you could experience chills after a hot flash. Cold shivers, sometimes known as cold flashes, are more common in some women than hot flashes.

Women experience hot flashes most frequently the year before and the year after their periods end. Hot flashes, however, can persist for up to 14 years following menopause, according to current research. Why hot flashes are so common during menopause is a mystery to medical professionals and scholars. Certain hot flashes can be avoided with medication, and you can attempt to control them when they do occur.

Tips:

Think about utilizing hormones: Discuss low-dose hormonal birth control with your doctor if you are still experiencing menstrual periods. This could alleviate some of your discomfort. Menopausal hormone therapy is an effective treatment for hot flashes and nocturnal sweats experienced by women who have gone through menopause. Hormone therapy for menopause carries several hazards. Find out from your doctor if it could be helpful. If menopausal hormone treatment is something you choose to undertake, take it for as little time as feasible at the lowest dose that relieves your symptoms.

Think about alternative medications: Should hormone therapy not be a possibility for you, consult your physician about prescription medications used to treat other conditions. Even if you don't have these specific medical conditions, some antidepressants, blood pressure medications, and epilepsy medications may help with hot flashes.

Monitor your bursts of heat: Jot down the things that give you hot flashes and make an effort to stay away from them. Foods that are spicy, alcohol, caffeine, stress, or being in a heated environment could all be triggers.

Sip some chilly water: When a hot flash is about to strike, have some icy water handy to sip from.

Remove an outer layer of clothing: Wear as many layers as you can.

Get a fan: If you can, keep a fan at work and turn on one beside your bed at night.

Inhale deeply: The moment a hot flash begins, try breathing deeply and slowly. Breathe deeply and slowly to signal your body to become calm and relaxed. Hot flashes may become shorter as a result.

Lose weight: Women who are overweight or obese may experience hot flashes more frequently. According to a recent study, hot flashes may get better with weight loss.

Vaginal infections problem

Vaginal issues, such as dry vagina, can arise or worsen throughout the menopausal period. Your vaginal tissue may become thinner and drier due to low estrogen levels. Itching, burning, and other pain or discomfort may result from this. Additionally, it may create little tears and wounds in your vagina during intercourse and make sex unpleasant. You are more susceptible to sexually transmitted

infections (STIs, or STDs) if you have vaginal
wounds or tears.

Tips:

Moisturizer for the vagina: Using an
over-the-counter vaginal moisturizer can help
maintain the lubrication of your vagina and
improve the comfort of your intercourse. This is
used every few days.

Lubrication for the vagina: Sex can be more
comfortable with the use of an over-the-counter
vaginal lubricant that is water-based. Either
before or during sex, you utilize this.

Prescription drugs: See your doctor about
further options for treating vaginal dryness,
such as hormonal birth control, menopausal
hormone therapy, or vaginally inserted
prescription estrogen creams, gels, or rings.
Find out more about menopausal remedies.
Speak with your doctor first because there are
hazards associated with any medications.

Irregular periods or bleeding

You may experience fewer or more periods.
They could be heavier or lighter, and they
might last more days or fewer. It's not always
the case that missing a few cycles indicates
you are entering the menopause or
perimenopause.

Tips:

Consult your physician to rule out any other
causes for your irregular periods, such as
pregnancy or a medical condition.
If you start bleeding or spotting after a year
without a period, you should also see your
doctor. Spotting or mild bleeding in women who
have gone through menopause may be related
to cancer or another major health issue.

Difficulty sleeping:

Many women going through menopause have
trouble staying asleep at night. Progesterone
deficiency might make it difficult to fall and
remain asleep. Hot flashes, which induce
sweating while you sleep, can also be brought

on by low estrogen levels. This is known as "night sweats" at times. Urinary problems are common in menopausal women, causing them to wake up multiple times during the night to go to the bathroom. You can also experience daytime fatigue that is unusual for you.

Tips:

Exercise: Engaging in regular physical activity is one of the finest strategies to achieve a restful night's sleep. However, you might have to exercise earlier in the day. You may become more awake if you exercise too soon before bed. Beginning a regular exercise routine during menopause may improve your mood, even if you have never done so before. Certain exercises, like yoga and stretching, have been shown in studies to potentially help reduce hot flashes.

Avoid eating, drinking, and smoking right before bed: Steer clear of heavy meals, smoking, and alcohol consumption just before bed. After noon, stay away from coffee.

Sip warm beverages: Before going to bed, consider having some warm liquid, like warm milk or caffeine-free tea.

Minimize screen time right before bed: Avoid using your computer, phone, or TV right before bed, especially in your bedroom. Your brain is told to wake up rather than sleep by the strong light from devices.

Adopt healthy sleeping practices: Maintain a cold, quiet, and dark bedroom. If you can, reserve your bedroom for sleeping and having sex.

Don't take a daytime sleep: Every day, try to go to bed and wake up at the same times.

Develop mental skills: Get up and do something soothing till you feel tired again if you wake up in the middle of the night and find it difficult to fall back again.

Speak with your nurse or physician: Your sleep issues may be serious, so discuss them with your physician or nurse. Sleep apnea and insomnia affect a lot of women. Improving chronic pain can also be aided by treating sleep issues.

Think about getting hot flash treatment: If your inability to sleep is being caused by your hot flashes, discuss treatment options with your physician or nurse. Usually, this will make you sleep better.

Address bladder issues: Consult a nurse or doctor about urinary tract treatment. Incontinence of the bladder or urine is not a typical aspect of aging. Certain therapies are effective.

Memory issues:

You could start to lose attention or get forgetful. Up to two thirds of women going through the perimenopause report experiencing memory loss or difficulty focusing. Memory loss and brain disorders, such as dementia and Alzheimer's disease, are not treated or prevented by menopausal hormone therapy. A recent study found that sleep deprivation and depression were associated with memory issues, but not estrogen levels.

Tips:

Get enough rest and exercise: maintain a nutritious diet, and abstain from smoking. This could help with memory.

Continue your social life: Join a club or group that focuses on your interests, like a quilting bee or a hiking club. Engaging in social interactions can help postpone memory loss and stave against illnesses like dementia and Alzheimer's.

Stay mentally active: Engaging in mental exercises such as crossword puzzles, attending classes, or picking up a new skill like learning a foreign language can help improve your memory and focus.

If amnesia or other mental health issues are interfering with your everyday life, see your doctor.

Urinary issues

During menopause, many women experience bladder or urine issues. Reduced estrogen levels could make the urethra weaker. It can be difficult for some women to contain their urination long enough to use the restroom. We refer to this as urge to urinate incontinence. Additionally, you could sneeze, cough, or laugh and end up leaking urine. Urinary stress incontinence is the term for this. The urge to urinate while sleeping has caused sleep disturbances for some women going through menopause. After menopause, urinary issues are not a typical aspect of aging and can be resolved.

Tips:

Depending on what caused the illness, treatment options for urine incontinence may include medication, physical therapy, the use of special medical devices, restricting or eliminating caffeine, or surgery.

You might experiment with urinary incontinence goods including pessaries, urethra caps, and pads if you experience pee leakage. Your urinary hole is covered by a urethra cap. It's reusable. A circular disk called a pessary is placed within your vagina to support your bladder. You can take it off, wash it, and put it back on yourself, but your doctor or nurse will fit you for your prosthesis.

See your physician or nurse about at-home treatments for incontinence of the urination. These could involve Kegel exercises, a unique type of exercise designed to strengthen your pelvic floor muscles. Losing weight may also be advised by your physician or nurse, as excess weight increases strain on the muscles around your bladder.

Mood swing:

You may experience periods of sobbing or irritability. Menopausal mood swings may be more likely to occur if you experienced depression or mood swings during your monthly periods after having birth. You may still have mood swings during menopause, even if you never had them during your monthly periods or after delivering birth. During this time, mood swings may also be caused by stress, family dynamics, or exhaustion. Mood swings and depression are not the same thing.

Tips:

Target getting seven or eight hours of sleep every night.

If you want to feel your best, get moving. Look for opportunities to exercise.

Try your best not to take on too many responsibilities. Seek out constructive methods to reduce your stress.

Become a member of a local or online support group for women experiencing menopause.

Discuss menopausal hormone therapy with your physician or nurse; it may be helpful for minor mood swings. Every medication, including menopausal hormone therapy, carries some risk. Menopause-related mood swings are typically not the same as depression, which is a distinct, severe condition that requires medical attention.

Anxiety and depression:

This is the period around menopause, when you are more susceptible to anxiety and despair. Menopausal symptoms, shifting hormones, or both could be the reason of this. The changes in your body or the loss of fertility may cause you to feel depressed or unhappy. Consult your physician if you're experiencing signs of anxiety or depression. For the treatment of anxiety or depression, your doctor can suggest medication, counseling, or both.

Tips:

Sleep: Make an effort to obtain enough rest. Most adult needs between seven and eight hours of sleep. Depression and sleep deprivation are related.

Exercise: Engage in physical activity for a minimum of half an hour most days of the week. Depression has been shown to improve with exercise. For ideas on how to get moving, check out our section on fitness.

Limit your alcohol intake: If you consume any alcohol at all, cut back on it. Women should limit their alcohol consumption to one drink per day and no more than seven drinks per week. Binge drinking is having four or more drinks in one go.

Feelings regarding sex changing

After menopause, some women experience a greater sense of comfort with their sexuality. Some people might not be as stimulated. If you are unpleasant or painful during sex, you might become less interested in it. Vaginal tissue that is thinner or drier may be the cause of this.

Tips:

There are safe over-the-counter and prescription solutions available to enhance vaginal lubrication if you are plagued by vaginal dryness. Find out more about your sexuality and the menopause.

Some menopausal symptoms, such as melancholy, anxiety, or insomnia, make some women less interested in having sex. If you're bothered by menopause symptoms, discuss potential therapies with your physician or nurse.

During menopause, many women find it beneficial to connect with encouraging family members or friends.

You are not alone if you are finding it difficult to discuss menopause. Keep that in mind. After a certain age, menopause affects all women.

Say that you would like to discuss about the menopause symptoms you are experiencing. Pose queries and share your personal narratives.

You may help your friends and family understand how menopause affects you by having conversations with them. They could have suggestions or ideas on how they can assist you.

Speak with your doctor or nurse if any of your menopausal symptoms are bothering you. When discussing treatments, you may touch on:

Your symptoms and the degree of your discomfort

Your age and health-related hazards for your health

Whether you have already received treatment similar to menopausal hormone therapy

Considering your past medical history and family history, determine if menopausal hormone therapy is a good option for you.

Whether or not you've gone through
post-menopause and, if so, when

Chapter Nine

Recipes for Menopause friendly meals

Here are a few recipes that are suitable for menopause that emphasize the use of nutrient-dense foods and promoting general wellbeing:

1.Salmon and Quinoa Bowl:

Ingredients:

- One cup of cooked quinoa

- One flaked salmon fillet, baked or grilled

- One cup of steaming broccoli

- Half an avocado, cut into slices

- One tablespoon of olive oil

- Lemon juice to taste

- To taste, add salt and pepper.

- Garnish with Fresh herbs, such as parsley or dill. Optional

Preparation:

- Steamed broccoli, sliced avocado, flaked salmon, and cooked quinoa should all be combined in a bowl.

- Pour in some lemon juice and olive oil. To taste, add salt and pepper for seasoning.

- Gently toss to mix in all the ingredients.

- If desired, garnish with fresh herbs.

Enjoy a nutrient-dense, omega-3-rich dinner that is served warm.

2. Salad with Chickpeas and Spinach:

Ingredients:

- 1 can (15 oz) of rinsed and drained chickpeas

- 2 cups of new, baby spinach

- Half a cup of cherry tomatoes

- 1 chopped cucumber

- 1/4 cup of crumbled feta cheese

- 2 teaspoons pure olive oil

- One-third cup balsamic vinegar

- 1 teaspoon Dijon mustard

- To taste, add salt and pepper.

Preparation:

- Chickpeas, baby spinach, cherry tomatoes, cucumber, and feta cheese should all be combined in a big bowl.

- Mix the olive oil, balsamic vinegar, Dijon mustard, salt, and pepper in a small bowl.

- Over the salad, drizzle with the dressing and gently mix to coat all the ingredients.

- Before serving, let the salad marinade
  for a few minutes.

Savor a revitalizing salad that is high in fiber, promotes digestive health, and offers vital minerals.

3. Tofu and Vegetable Stir-Fry

Ingredients:

- 1 cup of cubed firm tofu

- 2 cups of mixed veggies, including snap peas, carrots, bell peppers, and broccoli

- 1 tablespoon of sesame oil

- 2 teaspoons of soy sauce (low sodium)

- 1 tablespoon finely chopped fresh ginger

- 2 minced garlic cloves

- 1 tablespoon of optional sesame seeds

- Quinoa or brown rice for serving.

Preparation:

- Sesame oil should be stirred over medium to high heat in a wok or large pan.

- Stir-fry the tofu cubes until they turn golden brown.

- Add garlic, ginger, and mixed veggies.

- Stir-fry the veggies until they become crisp-tender.

- Add the soy sauce and mix everything until thoroughly covered.

- If desired, top with sesame seeds.

Serve over quinoa or brown rice for a filling, high-protein supper.

4. Berries and Greek Yogurt Parfait

Ingredients:

- 1 cup of plain Greek yogurt

- 3/4 cup of mixed berries, including raspberries, strawberries, and blueberries

- 1/4 cup low-sugar granola

- 1 tablespoon of honey (optional)

- Chopped nuts for garnish (walnuts, almonds).

Preparation:

- Place a layer of Greek yogurt in the bottom of a glass or bowl.

- Spread some mixed berries over the yogurt.

- Top the berries with a coating of granola.

- Until you reach the top of the container, keep going through the layers.

- If you'd like more sweetness, drizzle more maple syrup or honey over the top.

- Add chopped nuts as a garnish for extra crunch and good fats.

Savor a tasty, nutrient-rich yogurt parfait.

5. Avocado and Salmon Salad Wraps

Ingredients:

- 2 drained canned salmon fillets

- Mash one ripe avocado.

- Half a cup of cherry tomatoes

- 2 cups of mixed greens for salad

- Whole-grain tortillas

- Lemon dressing with olive oil

- To taste, add salt and pepper.

Preparation:

- Toss together canned salmon, cherry tomatoes, mashed avocado, and salad leaves in a bowl.

- Add a drizzle of lemon dressing and olive oil. Add pepper and salt for seasoning.

- After thoroughly mixing, pour mixture over whole-grain wrappers.

Enjoy a nutrient-dense, omega-3-rich supper that has been wrapped.

In order to maintain health throughout menopause, these recipes emphasize the use of nutrient-dense foods, lean meats, and entire ingredients. You are welcome to alter these

recipes to suit your dietary requirements and
personal preferences.

Conclusion

In conclusion, "Blooming through Menopause" is a valuable resource for women navigating the complexities of menopause, offering empowerment and information. This all-encompassing manual has navigated the physiological subtleties of this metamorphic stage, revealing the enormous influence of diet on general health. By stressing the need of a deliberate, well-balanced diet, the book gives its readers useful tools to help manage symptoms and adopt a better lifestyle.

Meal plans, recipes, and nutritional insights are more than just recommendations; they are a road map for building resilience, maintaining hormonal equilibrium, and maximizing well-being throughout menopause. The book acknowledges the special requirements of menopausal women and encourages the addition of foods high in nutrients, sources of omega-3 fatty acids, and thoughtful meal planning.

As the last chapter comes to a close, readers are motivated to start a journey of self-care and wellbeing in addition to being better informed.

"Blooming through Menopause" is a comprehensive method to enjoying this time of life with grace and vigor that goes beyond nutritional guidelines. Equipped with the knowledge and resources contained on these pages, women can view menopause as a chance for improved health and adaptability rather than as a barrier.